D1564774

Ultra HD Abs Workout

The Ultimate Guide to Getting Ultra-Abs

Table of Contents

Introduction

Before you become deeply involved in this book, I'm going to lay a few hard facts out for you right now. First, anyone can get abs. That's right, anyone. Even your 70-year-old grandfather, the fat postman who delivers your mail or the guy who works behind the checkout at McDonalds. They all have that ability.

Second, this can be achieved without the perceived need to do 1,000 sit-ups a day combined with running 100 miles a week and limiting your diet to salads. With the right information and guide to help you, you can still drink on weekends, eat those steak dinners you like and do ZERO cardio. It is really that simple.

So if it's that simple, then why doesn't your grandfather have six-pack abs? It would tempt your postman to deliver mail with his shirt off and display his glimmering abs, wouldn't he? And why doesn't your McDonalds order come with a side of six-pack abs? The only reason, and I do mean the only reason, is information. Although we all can have the desired body, few of us have the necessary information that could help us in our transformation.

That's where 'Ultra HD Abs Workout' comes into play. This book is a simple method to getting a six-pack. There are no tricks in here. No scams. You don't need to buy specialized equipment or supplements. As a reader, all you need to do is absorb the information and COMMIT.

Commitment is the most important aspect of achieving your dream physique. Knowing is only half the battle. As you read 'Ultra Abs HD Workout,' I want you to actually implement the tips that you read. Try them out, and experiment. Find the ones that are best for you. Because if you do, I promise you that you will throw away your large t-shirts within a matter of weeks as you won't need them anymore.

You'll have six new friends that you'll want to show off to the world.

'Ultra HD Abs Workout' can be broken down into two parts. The first part is diet. I hate to be the bearer of bad news but yes, what you eat has a huge impact on your ability to achieve a six-pack. This book is not about diet plans and calorie counting. But it will break down the main components of eating healthy and what to look out for.

The second section will cover the workouts. After providing a list of recommended workouts that you can try and how to properly do them, 'Ultra HD Abs Workout' will provide the actual routines. Combining core and ab workouts to create routines designed to give you, the reader, hot, new six-pack set of abs.

CHAPTER ONE – Two Steps to a Six-Pack

There are two important factors that you need to take control of in order to achieve a six-pack. The first and foremost is muscle development. The workouts that you do and making sure that you hit all the different sections of your abdominal muscles are the key. Without building muscle, there is no chance of having six-pack abs.

The second factor, which is equally important, is your diet.

Having abs and being able to develop six-pack abs are two completely different goals. Abs pertain entirely to the amount of FAT you in your stomach. You could have the hardest abdominal muscles in the world. But if you have too much fat on you, then it won't matter.

That's where diet comes into play. Diet is like a chisel that helps mold your abs once you've started building them. In 'Ultra HD Abs Workout,' we're going to concentrate on both factors; the workout and the diet. It's only when hitting them together that you can truly get an awesome six-pack.

CHAPTER TWO – The Diet

'Abs are made in the kitchen.' You have probably heard this cute, little phrase before. And although it may seem like a wishful thinking, it's actually a lot closer to the truth than you might want to believe.

But first, I just want to make something absolutely clear. You can't eat your way to a six-pack. That just isn't how muscle growth works. Even if you created the most perfectly balanced diet of all time for yourself, you still wouldn't have a six-pack. What you will have is just a flat stomach ripe for some sit-ups and ab development. But that's only half the battle. Working out and eating well are symbiotic. You need both to survive.

What I am going to talk about here are the three main food components you need to be aware of when honing a six-pack. You will often hear them referred to, as I will be from now on, as MACROS. These macros are *protein, carbohydrates or carbs* and *fats*. These three nutrients should feature in all meals in a balanced manner.

Unfortunately, each person is different. Because of this, 'Ultra HD Abs Workout' can't give you a guaranteed formula on how to mix the three. What it will do though is provide you with a rough percentage of how much of each macro you will need. And as you progress and learn, you can easily fiddle around with the amounts.

CALORIES

A quick note on calories: If you truly want to have a perfect six=pack you need to know how many calories per day you can consume without gaining unnecessary weight. Here are the calorie contents of the three macros:
Protein: 1 gram = 4 calories
Carbohydrates: 1 gram = 4 calories
Fats: 1 gram = 9 calories

You will need to use this basic module to discover how many calories you are consuming a day and how many of these calories adhere to your required macros.

PROTEIN

This is the grandfather of muscle development. If you think that you can get a six-pack without proper protein consumption, then you, my friend, are sadly mistaken. I hesitate to call it the most important macro because I believe that all three are equally important. But if there's one of them that has earned popularity, it is protein.

The key to eating protein when developing a six-pack is knowing what kinds of protein to eat. For optimum six-pack development, you need primarily eat *lean* proteins. These include *chicken, fish,* and *turkey.* These protein sources are very lean and contain very little fat, allowing you to eat as much as you like without having to worry too much about added weight.

But of course, you shouldn't eat as much as you want. There are proper proportions that you should be eating. The general rule for protein consumption is one gram of protein per pound of body weight per day. So if you weigh 130 pounds, you should aim to consume 130 grams of protein over the course of a day.

Now, assuming that you are eating a balanced meal that contains protein, carbs, and fats, then protein needs to account for a certain percentage of your daily calorie intake too. I recommend that the 35% of all calories consumed from the three macros should be from protein.

CARBOHYDRATES

I've felt pretty bad for carbs. They've gotten a really bad reputation in the past. People love to blame weight gain on carbs (and on fat for that matter too). But the truth is muscle growth and thus six -pack development is impossible without carbs. Carbs provide the energy that your body needs in order to operate. Your muscles quite literally look to the carbs you eat to facilitate growth. Where protein is the cement used to hold the bricks on the wall, carbs are the worker that actually puts it all together.

So why do people hate carbs? The primary reason is that carbs are a blanket term used for a variety of food groups. The most well-known is sugar. Sugar loves to live inside carbs. The two go together like peas and carrots. Whether you're drinking soda or eating cake, these are bad carbs. But carbs nonetheless. The key here is to know which ones to eat.

When working on your six-pack, please stick to simple carbs. These are carbs that haven't been artificially developed and come naturally from the earth and thus, don't contain any added sugar. I recommend eating mainly potatoes (normal and sweet) and rice (brown especially). Yes, you can eat bread and pasta too but it's important to note that these both have been artificially made. Depending on the brand or where you buy it from, they contain added sugar. So be wary.

But how much to eat? As you are working on your six-pack here, we don't want to go too heavy on the carbohydrate level. I would recommend that 45% of your total daily calories from the macros come from simple carbs. This may seem like a lot but if you're working out properly, then it really is the optimum.

FATS

Fats, like carbs, have a pretty bad reputation too. And like carbs, it's for the same reason. So many different and unhealthy, foods fall into the fat category (and it doesn't help that the word itself is a synonym for being overweight).

First, let's list the four major types of fats. There's monounsaturated, polysaturated, trans and unsaturated. Don't worry, these names aren't too important. What is important is being able to recognize them.

The two types that you want to look for are monounsaturated and polyunsaturated. These are the good fats, the ones that work for, not against you. You can find these in avocados, nuts, peanut butter (organic), and fatty fish such as salmon. When I talk about eating fat this is what I'm concentrating on.

The fats you really want to avoid are trans fats and saturated fats. Trans fats are found primarily in oily food like chips, burgers, and anything deep fried. You know is bad to eat but with trans fat make food taste so good that it would be hard for you not to consume them. The other is saturated fat. Similar to trans in how bad it can be for you, this one is found in creamy foods like butter, cheeses, and milk. Building a six-pack is primarily about having as little fat over your abdomen as possible. Thus, avoid these two fat groups like plague.

Now when eating fats, you're going to want to cover the remainder of your macro intake. You have 20% left to use, these should go to fats. Be careful though. The reason that fats are so dangerous is that they contain twice the calories of proteins and carbs. So when you're eating them, make sure to keep the portions small.

These are the three main nutrients you need to look for, proteins, fats, and carbs. When eaten at a proper ratio and in conjunction with a proper workout regime, they work together and help the body grow. Try them out, mix them up. Find out what combination best works for you and your body type because the next step is working out.

But before that, I need to mention one final food group that you must, under all circumstances, stay away from.

SUGAR

This one is a doozy and the number one enemy in creating a six -pack. Even if you eat all your other macros in a perfect balance, sugar threatens to ruin them all. And more often than not, it does more than threaten. Sugar is like your cruel ex who will stop at nothing to lure you back to what seems like a pleasure town only to destroy your life.

The issue with sugar is that it loves to hide. Some sugars are obvious. Candy, sweets, chocolates. Everyone knows that these are chock full of the good stuff. I am saying this with absolute conviction; do not eat these if you want a six-pack. Yes, you can start spoiling yourself over time when you learn more about your body and what you can and can't eat. But for now, as you are still learning, avoid these sweets like the devil.

But there are also the hidden sugars that you don't even know about. Bread is a big one. This is a baked product sold in stores which is full of sugar to give it a sweeter taste. Even fruits. Most fruits contain more sugar than candy. I'm not saying don't eat fruits. I'm saying don't order a juice and think that you're slimming down because it's the exact opposite.

And there's also the added sugar. Any product that you buy in a can or packaging will have added sugar. The average can of peeled tomatoes contains six grams of added sugar alone. Be wary when you buy packaged food and always check the label.

WATER RETENTION

This is something that is rarely talked about but is invaluable information when it comes to getting ripped. Sometimes our diet will be on point, our workouts will be massive and out body fat percentage will be at an all-time low. But for some reason, you will still look puffy. You know the abs are there but they aren't showing. This is most likely due to water retention.

Some foods store water easier than others. As a result, the cells in our body appear to be 'puffing' out, making us look sluggish and fat when in reality this is just excess water. Now, I wouldn't be too concerned about this occurrence. It's not permanent and can easily be managed. You just need to know what foods can retain water.

Salts are a big one. The saltier your food is, the more likely that it is to retain extra water. Some dairy products, such as milk and cheese, also have a similar effect. Now, it's important to note that I'm not telling you to give up these foods entirely, just to be wary. If you are noticing that you feel bloated after certain meals, target what causes that feeling and try eliminating it from your diet. You might be shocked by the results.

I promise that if you eat well, a six-pack will come twice as easy for you than if you don't. In fact, if you balance your macros properly, you can even achieve a hard six-pack without the aid of cardio exercise. Diet is really that important.

CHAPTER THREE – The Lifestyle

Although this is going be a short chapter, it's also one of the most important. I'm going to use it to talk about lifestyle; more specifically, your lifestyle and how you can take simple steps in your day-to-day activities to better increase your odds of having a six-pack.

I know you're probably mad at me. I did promise that you wouldn't have to do cardio six times a week. And I did promise that you could keep eating those steak dinners you seem to love so much. And the truth is, you can. Hell, you can have pizza every night of the week if you are living the proper lifestyle.

Now, what do I mean by this?

The first point obviously pertains to your diet. I addressed it pretty specifically in the previous chapter. But it still warrants a small mention here. My point, to put simply, is to try and keep your diet balanced. Can you have pizza every night of the week? Of course, you can. It just means that your other meals are going to have to be smaller and macro (protein and carbs) heavy. Can you have a doughnut at the end of the week? I don't see why not. As long as your other meals throughout the day have been balanced.

That's what I mean when I say balance. You can have the bad but make sure you know why it is bad for you and what you can do to counter-act it.

But a proper lifestyle also refers to the physical aspects of your life. How much physical exercise do you do a week? Be honest now. No, you don't need to do massive amounts of cardio. Yes, you can watch Netflix all day. But in the long run, that's just going to make the journey harder for you. You bought 'Ultra HD Abs Workout,' because you want to change. It begins with lifestyle.

Changing your lifestyle means looking for opportunities to be physically active throughout the day. Walk to the local store rather than drive. Buy a bike and ride to work rather than getting a bus. Walk to buy your lunch rather than ordering in every day. You don't even have to break a sweat. Just the constant action of physical movement will help put your body into fat burning mode. The less fat, the more chance there is of having a six-pack set of abs.

ALCOHOL

When talking about lifestyle, alcohol always warrants a brief mention. It's probably the thing I'm asked about most. Can you drink and still have a six-pack? The short answer is yes as long as you keep it in moderation. Balance applies to everything here, it's what I've been spouting in the first few pages and will continue to spout for the remainder of them. Can you drink every night? No (regardless of your life goals, I wouldn't recommend this). Can you get absolutely blasted on a Friday night without worrying too much? Hell, yeah you can.

Like diet, it's just important to know what alcoholic drinks are better and why the bad ones are bad. When I drink, I stick to spirits. Particularly gin and vodka, these two are low on calories and when mixed with soda water are perfectly legitimate drinks to have without feeling guilty. What makes them dangerous is when you start mixing them with soda. Remember, soda is almost all sugar, the number one cause of weight gain.

We then get to our beers and wines. These are both pretty bad for you. Where wine is filled with sugar, beer is filled with empty carbs. Neither is great for you. But again, you can have a night of the week where you drink nothing but beer. Just make sure that the week leading up to this was filled with healthy eating and workouts. The same goes for wine.

I'm not trying to tell you what you can and can't eat or drink. I'm saying that you can eat and drink everything and anything. Just keep it balanced. That is the real key to getting a six-pack.

Lifestyle Tip: Swap sodas for water. Water is essential for transporting and metabolizing the macros that we eat every day. We should drink at least two liters of water a day.

CHAPTER FOUR – The Core

I'm going to take a second here to talk about the core.

I'm sure you've heard people talk about core strength a lot and how important it is. But you've probably never really figured out what it is; or more importantly how it relates to getting a six-pack. Having a strong core is the number one step you must take to achieve this. A six-pack and a strong core are, in a sense, one and the same.

Now, can you have a six pack with a weak core? Sure you can. But do you want to? Hell no. Luckily this is pretty hard to do anyway. Most ab and core exercises overlap to a certain degree, even to the point where it's near impossible to work one without working the other.

I am going to list a series of my favorite core workouts below. Although a lot of these workouts also engage abdominal development, they do focus primarily on core strength.

Lifestyle Tip: Eat your greens. Although they don't fall into any of the macro groups, make sure to have a healthy serving of greens with every meal. My personal favorite is broccoli.

THE WORKOUTS

The Plank

This is the grandfather of the core workout. If you can only do one core exercise, make it this one. It's easy to do, effective and can be done with minimal equipment. All you need is time and space.

Muscles Targeted: Obliques

Repetition Range: Hold for a minimum of one minute or as long as possible.

1) Lie face down with your chest and face pressed up against the floor.
2) Push up so that you are supporting yourself with your toes and forearms. Your forearms running flat along the ground while bent directly below your shoulders.
3) Make sure to keep your body and most importantly, your back, straight.

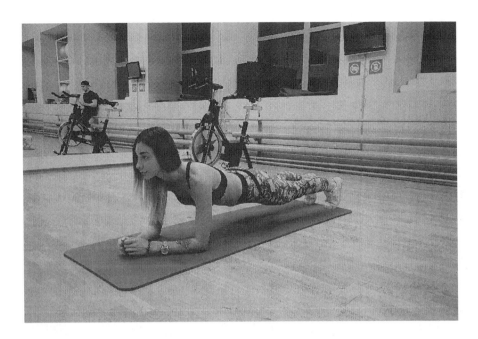

Variations:

Military Plank

This is a good one for when you become bored of planks. It puts a little more pressure on your oblique muscles while the added push up motion helps engage the serratus and transverse abdominis.

Muscles Targeted: Serratus, Obliques, Transverse Abdominis

Repetition Range: 10-15 full movements. This is a good fat burner so don't be afraid to do a few more if you can.

1) Get into the same position as you would in an ordinary plank.

2) Once balanced, ensure that you keep your back straight, push yourself up to the flat of your hands so that your elbows are no longer bent. Keep your hands by your side.
3) Next, drop back down to your elbows. Hold for a second before going back up.

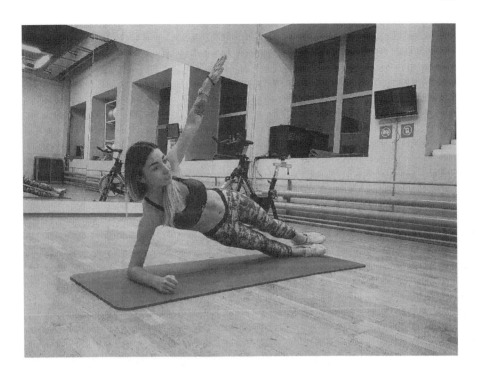

Weight Switch

This is a fun variation of the standard plank. I would suggest this for those who need to plank for several minutes at a time. The added use of weights really targets growth of the oblique muscles.

Muscles Targeted, Serratus, Obliques,

Repetition Range: 10 switches to either side.

1) Select a small dumbbell. *Nothing too heavy. A weight you can do for thirty reps of curls with.
2) Get into a plank position, put the dumbbell just within reach of your right hand.

3) Maintain balance on your left forearm and reach for the dumbbell with your right hand, drop it underneath your chest.

4) Next, shift your balance to your right forearm, lift the dumbbell with your left hand and move it to your left side. Drop it just within reach.

5) Pause for a second before repeating the action, this time moving the weight to your right side.

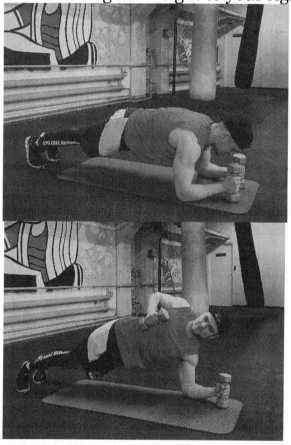

Renegade Rows

This has got to be my favorite core workout. The primary reason is that it's so simple to execute and with the addition of weights, when done properly, really tears at the core.

Caution: This is a tough exercise. A strong back is recommended before trying.

Muscles Targeted: Serratus, Obliques, Transverse Abdominis

Repetition Range: Between 8-10 altogether. This one is concentrated on muscle building. A higher rep range is pointless.

1) Select two heavy dumbbells. *a weight that you can curl 6-8 times.
2) Place the dumbbells on the floor, roughly shoulder width apart.
3) Grab a hold of the two dumbbells, position yourself as if you were doing a pushup.
4) Now, using one dumbbell for support and balance, lift the other up to your side. Making sure to keep your back straight and core engaged. Do not turn your body as you do this.
5) Hold weight parallel to side for two seconds before placing the dumbbell back on the floor.
6) Alternate the movement with the other dumbbell.

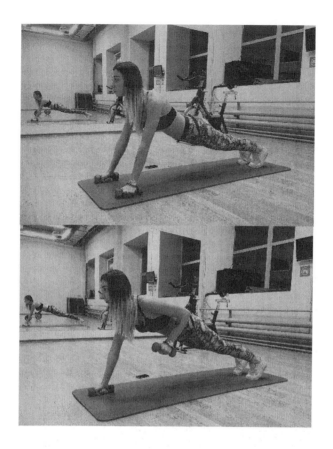

Cables

Cable core workouts can be convenient in a busy gym with minimal floor space. They do have their drawbacks though. Unless done properly, they don't isolate the core and can easily be cheated by the lazy gym goers. However, I enjoy doing them as they don't require you to lie down on the ground.

There are three main ways to utilize the cables in a cow workout. They are listed below.

Muscles Targeted: Serratus, Obliques

Repetition Range: Keep this one heavy and to about 6 repetitions on each side.

Variations

Standing Russian Twist

1) Connect a handle attachment to the cable machine and adjust so that the handle is in line with your belly button.
2) Place both feet firmly on the ground and away from the machine. You should be approximately arm's length from the handle, with the attachment dangling just behind your back.
3) Keep your feet firmly placed; turn your body backward to take hold of the handle attachment.
4) Then, make sure to use only your abdominal muscles, spin body forward, pull the handle with you. Elbows are to be kept straight.
5) Once facing forward, slowly turn back until the handle attachment is back to its original position. Repeat.

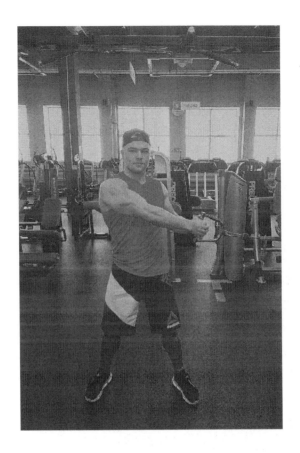

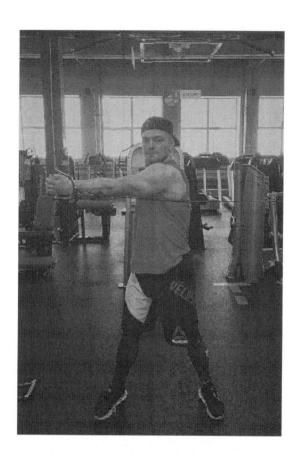

Standing Wood Chop

1) Connect the handle attachment to the highest possible position on the cable machine.
2) Stand in a similar position as if you were doing a standard Russian twist.
3) Next, take the handle with both hands, pull down in one motion across the front of your body.
4) Make sure that your back and arms are both straight, swing the handle like a large sword. Keep core tight.

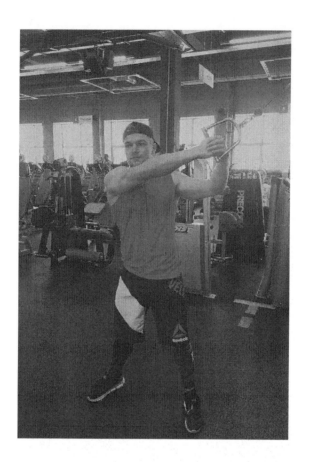

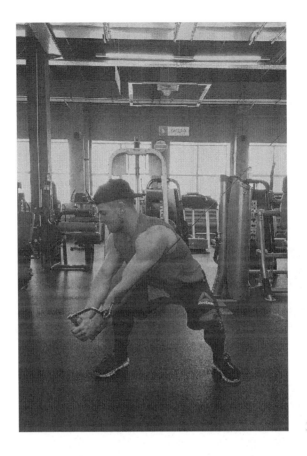

Standing Cable Lift

1) Connect the handle attachment to the lowest possible point on the cable machine.
2) Stand in a similar position as if you were doing a Russian twist.
3) Next, taking the handle with both hands and pull upwards in one motion, making sure to keep arms and back straight as if swinging a golf club.
4) Make sure to keep your core tight.

Lifestyle Tip: Don't be fooled by 'no sugar' products. Although they don't put on weight directly, artificial sweeteners create fat deposits in the body which literally makes it easier for you to gain fat.

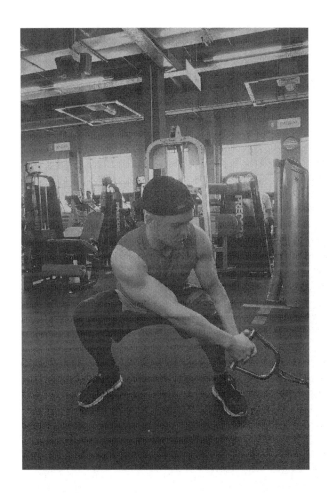

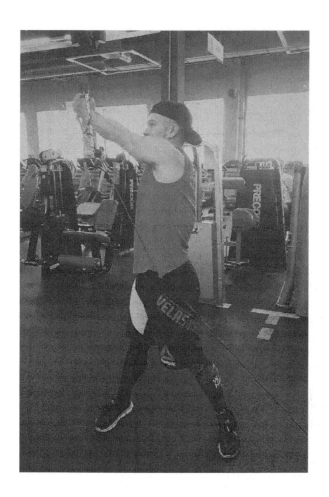

Ab-Roller

This is a pretty important core workout and one I would highly recommend to anyone who can actually do it. Like the plank, it fully isolates and engages your core muscles. However, the added movement engages the rectus abdominis, thus, encouraging faster muscle growth than a standard plank would.

Tip: If you don't have an ab-roller, use a skateboard instead. It works equally as well.

Caution: This is a tough exercise. A strong back is recommended before trying.

Muscles Targeted: Rectus Abdominis, Obliques

Repetition Range: 10-12 full movements. This will get easier over time and once the Bosu Ball becomes a standard. I would suggest pausing horizontal to the ground to put extra pressure on the core.

1) Kneel on the floor, take the ab-roller with both hands, placing it in front you.
2) Remaining on your knees, slowly roll forward, gripping the ab-roller by its handles. Make sure to keep the core engaged as you move to fully extend your elbows.
3) Once you are out flat, stomach hovering above the ground, elbows extended; pause for as long as possible before pulling yourself back to a kneeling position.

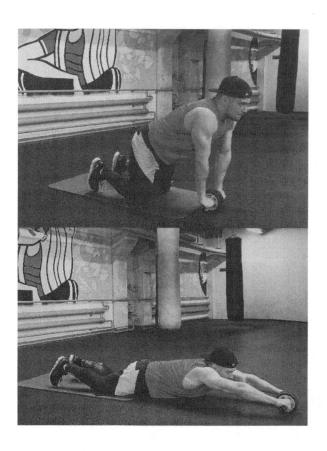

Variations

Barbell Ab-Roller

This one is for a gym goer who doesn't have access to an ab-roller. Not all gyms have them. The result is the same; it's just the method that varies slightly.

1) Take a standard barbell and attach round weight plates to either side. Weight not important.
2) Position self as if you were about to do an ab-roll exercise. This time, however, have the barbell with attached weights sitting in front of you within reach.
3) Grip the barbell with both hands, arms shoulder width apart.
4) Like an ab-roll, simply roll self forward, making sure the back is kept flat and knees remain where they are.
5) Hold for as long as possible before pulling self-back to kneeling position.

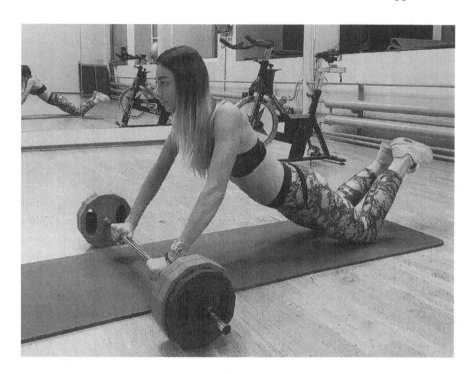

Bosu Ball Ab-Roller

When a workout becomes stale or too easy, you should be looking for ways to change or improve on the current formula. This Bosu Ball Ab-Roller is a perfect example of adding an extra degree of difficulty to a workout.

1) Kneel on the center of a bosu ball. Making sure you are balanced.
2) Hold the ab-roller as normal, perform a standard ab-roll. Knees remaining in place on the bosu-ball.
3) Keep core engaged the whole time. Be careful not to use arms or back when pulling self back to a kneeling position.

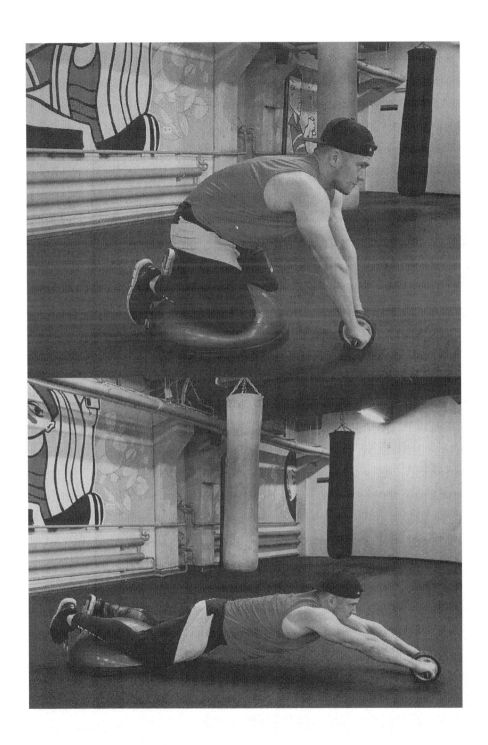

CHAPTER FIVE – The Abdominals

Here we go to the main event. If you've read this far, then you truly are interested in getting those washboard abs. So for that, I thank and congratulate you.

It's important to note that the abdominals aren't one single muscle. They are made up of several different muscle groups. They include:

- ***Rectus Abdominis***: These are what most people think of when imagining a six-pack. They run from the sternum to the pelvic bone, covering the front and centre of the stomach.
- ***Transverse Abdominis:*** Hidden from sight, these muscles run underneath your obliques, wrapping around your spine like a girdle.
- ***Obliques***: These guys frame the side of your abdominals, acting like a frame on either side of your rectus abdominis.
- ***Intercostals***: A pretty underrated muscle, it is located between the sides of the ribcage.
- ***Serratus.*** Located between the front of your abs and lats, they are most visible during twisting motions.

These are all important and all need to be worked equally.

You don't need to remember the names. You really just need an idea of where each muscle group is located and where each one separates from. This will allow you to hit all of them when do you the exercises. Lifestyle Tip: Try to cut back on snacking. Snacking can mess with your metabolism. I recommend four square meals a day.

THE WORKOUTS

The Crunch

The original abdominal workout. Although it's a little dated, it's still handy to know about. The further beauty of this exercise is its variation. Literally, every change of angle or weight added can target your abs in a different way. I'm going to list a few here but I encourage you to try and find as many variants of this workout as you can.

Muscles Targeted - Rectus Abdominis

Repetition Range: As mentioned, these are fast-twitch muscle exercise. For all crunch exercises, keep the range between 12 and 15 reps.

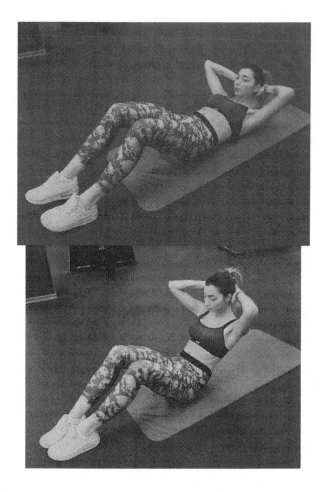

Variations

Cross-Body Crunch

Muscles Targeted: Rectus Abdominis, Obliques, Intercostals

1) Lie on the flat of your back, knees bent, feet flat on the floor.
2) Hold hands behind head, making sure elbows stick out.

3) Curl body forward while bringing your right knee up and toward your left shoulder, across your chest.
4) Touch your knee to your elbow, make sure to contract your ab muscles at the same time.
5) Repeat with the opposite side.

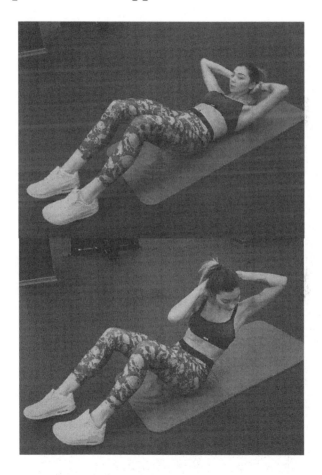

Cross Crunch

Muscles Targeted: Rectus Abdominis, Obliques, Intercostals

1) Lie on the flat of your back, knees bent, feet flat on the floor. Hands by your side.
2) Curl body forward as if doing a standard crunch.
3) When halfway up, reach out with your right hand and tap your left knee.
4) Lay back down.
5) Repeat this movement with the opposite side.

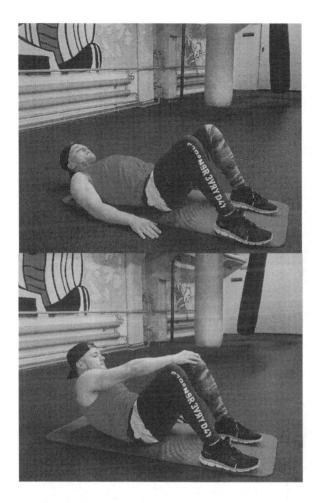

Decline Crunch

Tip: Try different movements while in the decline position. Don't just stick to the standard crunch.

Muscles Targeted: Rectus Abdominis,

1) Locate a bench that goes into the decline position.
2) Repeat standard crunch.

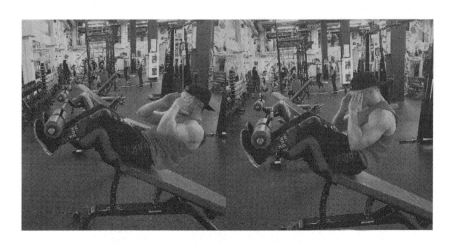

Exercise Ball Crunches

Muscles Targeted: Rectus Abdominis, Intercostals

1) Find an exercise ball that will support your weight.
2) Sit on the ball so that feet are placed firm and flat on the ground.
3) Lean back slowly, ensure that you remain perfectly steady.
4) Once leaning back as far as is comfortable, sits yourself up, engaging abdominal muscles as you do.

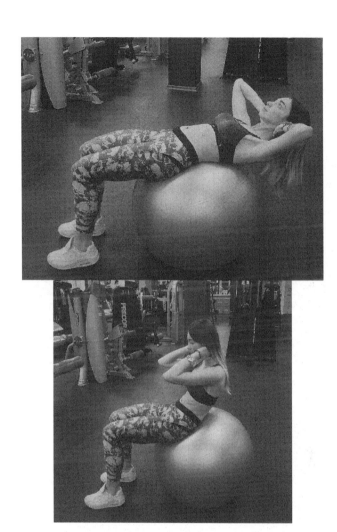

Weighted Sit-Ups

The most simple and well known of all abdominal workouts (barring the crunch, of course). This one is great for pure muscle development. I always do it, just as a simple way to wear out my rectus abdominis after or even before a workout.

Tip: Make sure to keep your movements nice and slow with this one. Faster movements tend to disengage core.

Muscles Targeted: Rectus Abdominis

Repetition Range: As there is weight involved in this one, I would keep the reps to 10-12.

1) Select a weight. It could be a dumbbell, weight plate or medicine ball.
2) Lie flat on your back, knees bent with your feet flat on the ground.
3) Hold the weight firmly on your stomach, hold slightly closer to your chin, slowly sit up.
4) Make sure to keep your feet flat and back straight for the entirety of the motion.

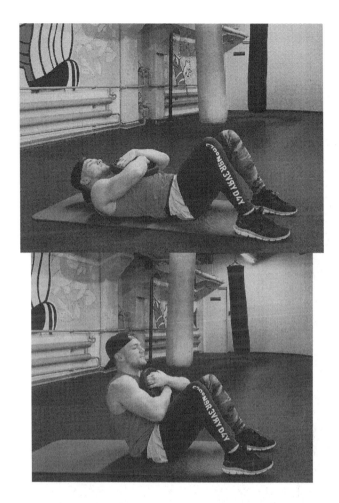

Russian Twists

Like the weighted sit up, this one is pretty stock standard. It's a little more advanced than the basic weighted sit up because the extra twisting motion puts pressure on the obliques and intercostals.

Lifestyle Tip: Flex your abdominal muscles as much as possible, even when juts sitting at work. The constant work keeps them active.

Muscles Targeted: Rectus Abdominis, Obliques, Intercostals

Repetition Range: Like the weighted sit up, this should be done at a 10-12 rep range. One rep should be a full rotation to both sides.

1) Select an appropriate weight. This can be either a medicine ball or a weight plate.
2) Lie flat on the floor, feet flat on the floor.
3) Holding the weight in your hands, sit up so that your body creates a V-Shape.
4) Keeping slightly bent, twist body down and to the right side. Ensure that feet remain planted on the floor.
5) Hold for a second before twisting back to the other side, making sure that body remains in the V-Shape.

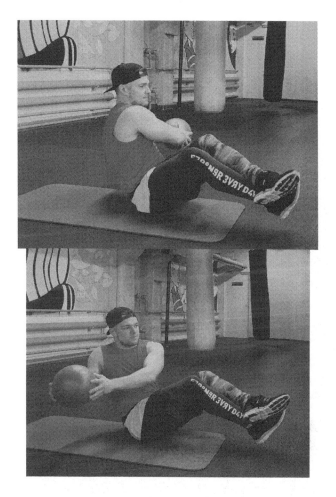

Variations

Russian Ball Passes

This is a tricky one but handy for further engaging a few extra muscles that you don't get to from the basic Russian Twist.

Tip: Try and drop the ball into the hand rather than pass. The dropping motion forces the obliques to engage as they struggle to hold up the added weight.

Muscles Targeted: Rectus Abdominis, Obliques, Serratus, Intercostals, Transverse Abdominis

Repetition Range: I like to think of it as more of a fat burner than the other core workouts. Therefore, push the reps up to 30 full passes.

1) Select an appropriate medicine ball.

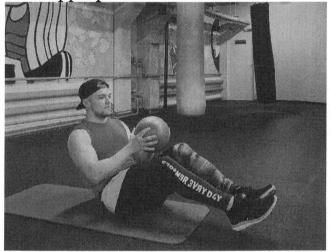

2) Put yourself in the same position as a standard Russian Twist.
3) Now, raise your feet off the ground so that your entire body is in a V-Shape and only your bottom rest on the floor. Knees still bent.
4) Holding the medicine ball in your right hand, pass it over your right thigh, underneath your left thigh, taking it with your left hand.
5) Then, in a continuous motion, pass the ball over your left thigh, under your right thigh, taking the ball back with your right hand.
6) Continue this motion.

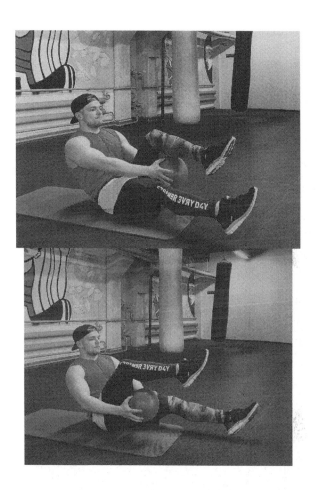

Leg Raises

This is a pretty well-known one too. It's convenient because it can be done literally anywhere, anytime. It's also good for targeting the Transverse Abdominis, a muscle that gets the least amount of work.

Note: I'll be outlining the basic technique here. This exercise also works in a hanging position and on a variety of different benches. I suggest trying them all to find which works best for you.

Muscles Targeted: Rectus Abdominis, Intercostals, Transverse Abdominis

Repetition Range: These are similar to crunches in the way they work your abs. Keep the rep range between 12 and 15 for all.

1) Lie on the flat of your back. Leg's straight, arms by your side.
2) With your legs held together, keep them straight as you raise them as high as they will go.
3) Keep the motion slow and steady as you bring it to completion, finish them flat on the floor.
4) Feel free to add a weight to your legs if this is too easy for you.

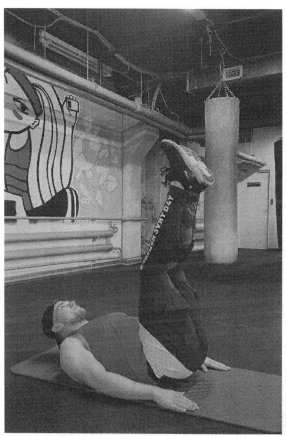

Variations

Leg Pull Ins

1) Position yourself similar to a standard leg raise.
2) Now, rather than raising your legs straight and flat, bend your knees as you pull them in tight to your chest.
3) Make sure to contract the abdominal muscles as you do.

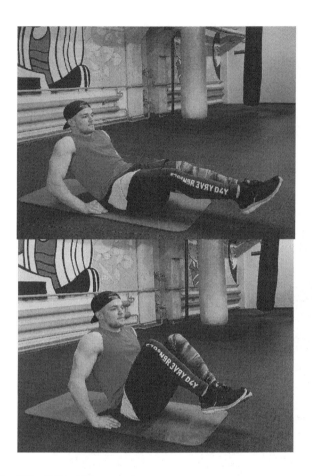

Jack Knife Sit Up

1) Lie flat on your back with your arms held straight back behind your head. Your legs straight on the floor.
2) Now, bend your waist into a sit up while simultaneously raising your legs and hands from the floor.
3) Your hands should meet your ankles in a V-Shape above the centre of your body.
4) Exhale and lower yourself back down to the floor.

Bottom Ups

1) Lie flat on the ground, your legs extended out and arms by your waist.
2) Tuck your knees into your chest then follow this by pushing them upwards and toward the sky.

3) The finished movement will have you resting on your shoulder blades as your feet point vertically in the air.
4) Make sure to keep your abdominals contracted during the entire movement.

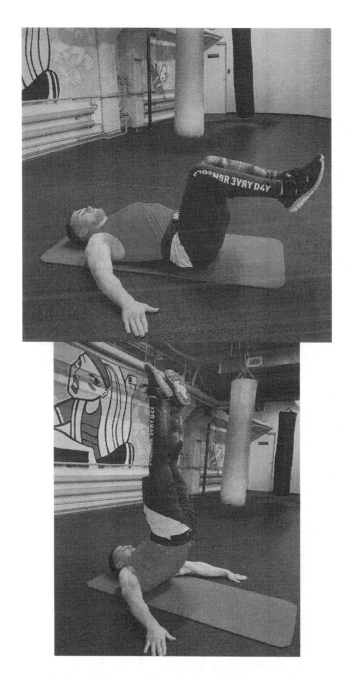

Scissor Kicks

1) Lie flat on the ground, your legs extended out and arms by your waist.
2) Raises both feet several inches off the ground while contracting your abdominals slightly and tucking your chin into your chest
3) Kick your feet, one up and one down, in a scissor motion and make sure to keep them elevated off the ground.
4) This is a wear-and-tear exercise – go until you can't anymore.

CHAPTER SIX - The Routines

You have a basic understanding of diet. You have a list and explanations of the best exercises. Now it's time to actually put them to work.

You might be tempted to just do one or two sets of every single exercise until you tire out. Then pick it up again the next day and continue like that. Sure, by doing this, you are working your abs pretty hard and yes, you will start to see the result. But they won't be conclusive and will most likely come out lopsided. What do I mean by this?

Remember how I listed the different sections of your abdominals? Each of these has its own muscle. If you just run through the exercises as you feel like it, you risk working one particular section more than the other. Although the odds of you coming out looking like Quasimodo are slim, there's no point risking it.

As a result, I've written up three routines that target all the muscles that make up a six-pack. Each day is designed to impact your abdominals differently, so make sure you don't skip one.

Do one routine every 2-3 days. Make sure to rotate them evenly. And stick to the repetition ranges recommended in the workout descriptions.

Lifestyle Tip: Create a situation where you have to walk every day, even if it's just ten minutes down the road to get a coffee. You'd be surprised by the results.

ROUTINE ONE

The Basics

This is a nice and simple routine to get you into gear. The exercises here are non-complex movements that are designed to build muscles while stabilizing the core.

Do three sets of each in the order listed. And unless specified, stick to the rep range provided in the workout description.

Lifestyle Tip: The skipping rope is probably the easiest way to burn fat. A ten minute skip equates to almost thirty minutes of cardio.

Muscles Worked: Rectus Abdominis, Obliques, Intercostals, Transverse Abdominis, Serratus

1) PLANK
2) RUSSIAN TWISTS
3) LEG RAISES *I would suggest adding a weight where possible for that extra burn.
4) WEIGHTED CRUNCHES *this is added here to really work and wear down your rectus abdominis before the final exercise.

5) MILITARY PLANKS *do as many as possible here. At this point, reaching the desired rep range should be near impossible.

ROUTINE TWO

Oblique Blast

As the name suggests, this routine is designed to primarily target the obliques. After the rectus abdominis, I think the obliques are the most important and definitive muscle in having a six-pack. It's important to show them some extra love every once in a while.

Lifestyle Tip: As this one involves muscle building, I would suggest a slightly higher protein/carb intake on this day and fewer fats.

Muscles Worked: Muscles Worked: Rectus Abdominis, Obliques, Intercostals, Transverse Abdominis, Serratus

1) WEIGHT SWITCH PLANKS *don't be afraid to increase the weight when you think you are ready.
2) STANDING CABLE RUSSIAN TWISTS
3) SCISSOR KICKS *this is placed here to give you a small reprieve before going into the harder stuff.
4) RUSSIAN BALL PASS
5) CROSS BODY CRUNCH

ROUTINE THREE

Advanced Stabilizing

I'm a big proponent of training core, often at the expense of targeting specific abdominal muscles. This routine is a perfect combination of hardcore training while still making sure to hit the rectus abdominis.

Lifestyle Tip: Don't be afraid to spoil yourself a little after a workout. A heavy workout leaves the body working extra hard to make up for the energy lost. Post workouts can be the best time to 'cheat' a little.

Muscles Worked: Muscles Worked: Rectus Abdominis, Obliques, Intercostals, Transverse Abdominis, Serratus

1) AB ROLLER *don't be afraid to mix it up with a Bosu Ball if this becomes too easy.
2) RENEGADE ROWS
3) JACK KNIFE SIT UPS
4) DECLINE CRUNCHES *weights can be added if you feel so inclined.
5) WEIGHTED CRUNCHES *placed at the end to ensure that this workout feels complete. Make sure to take these extra slow.

Final Note

These are but three of hundreds of possible workout combinations. I chose these three for their variation in exercises and what each routine aims to do. However, please take note that all three target all the muscle groups needed to get a six-pack. This is important.

I encourage you to mix and match some of the exercises now that you know them. But when you do, make sure that each muscles group are targeted at least once.

And finally, enjoy your new six-pack. You've earned it.

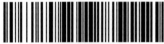

Made in the USA
Lexington, KY
23 July 2017